THE MEDICAL ASSISTANT'S SURVIVAL GUIDE

Inez Gregory

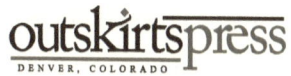

The opinions expressed in this manuscript are solely the opinions of the author and do not represent the opinions or thoughts of the publisher. The author has represented and warranted full ownership and/or legal right to publish all the materials in this book.

The Medical Assistant's Survival Guide
All Rights Reserved.
Copyright © 2016 Inez Gregory
v2.0

This book may not be reproduced, transmitted, or stored in whole or in part by any means, including graphic, electronic, or mechanical without the express written consent of the publisher except in the case of brief quotations embodied in critical articles and reviews.

Outskirts Press, Inc.
http://www.outskirtspress.com

ISBN: 978-1-4787-7010-7

Outskirts Press and the "OP" logo are trademarks belonging to Outskirts Press, Inc.

PRINTED IN THE UNITED STATES OF AMERICA

Contents

Preface 1
How It All Began 4
The Doctor is in the House 6
Formal Training or On-the-Job Training? 8
Not Enough Hands To Go Around 11
Personality and Time Management 13
Notation! Notation! Notation! 15
Weighty Matters 17
Why Medical Assisting? 19
Take a Breather! 21
Mum is Definitely Not The Word 23
Administrative or Clinical? 25
Why Certification? 28
You Get As Much As You Give 31
Health Concerns 33
Is Medical Assisting Enough? 34
Good Evening Professors, Administrators,
Distinguished Guests and My Fellow Medical Assistants! ... 36
AFTERWORD AND ACKNOWLEDGEMENTS 39

Preface

SOME PEOPLE KNOW in the beginning what they want to be when they grow up. I never thought I had an aptitude for the medical field. I only know the commercial I saw one day made the medical field seem very rewarding. It was actually about a nursing assistant. When I went to gather information at the college that sponsored the commercial, the admissions officer said I should consider being a medical assistant. I had never heard of medical assisting. What does one do as a medical assistant?

I was simply told that if I chose the medical assisting major, I would be indispensable in the doctor's office. Wow! What about the hospital? I had to change my whole way of thinking and get used to the idea of being in school an additional year, pursuing a degree instead of a certificate. The whole thing sounded intriguing. I decided to go for it. The decision would lead me on a life-changing journey that would compare with nothing I ever encountered. I will forever reap the benefits of such a multi-faceted career.

I've met individuals from all walks of life and worked in various medical specialties. I've seen medical miracles and I've weathered crushing patient prognoses. I've seen brand new patients only hours old in receiving blankets and I've lost precious friends who were great grandparents.

If you love humanity, you'll love medical assisting. It's not easy but anything worth having is rarely a piece of cake.

This book is written to help you on your medical assisting career path. Whether you are certified or uncertified or even if you are thinking of another career option in the medical arena, this book will give you insight into the world of the doctor's office. The writing of this book has been therapeutic and cathartic. We stand presently as the sum of our past experiences. If I had to do it all over again, I wouldn't change a thing. I would choose to keep the experiences the same-mistakes and all-for it is the mistakes that lead to the path of perfection. Compassion reigns in the medical industry so if you don't have a heart-don't start.

There are many texts used to instruct students on how to be a medical assistant. However, I have yet to encounter a book written from the perspective of a seasoned professional. There is the classroom and then there is the "real world" doctor's office.

What I have done here is reach from my experience as a certified medical assistant to help those of you who either have or have not graduated from an accredited medical assisting program who are pursuing a career in medical assisting. Even if you are only beginning to consider a degree in the medical assisting arena, I hope the advice given helps not only the intended audience but also all members of the allied health professions.

I have a very rewarding career. Some days are incredibly

tough, but I know at the end of the day, there is nothing else I would rather be doing.

   Inez Gregory, C.M.A.

How It All Began

I WASN'T ONE of the geniuses who knew from the first breath on Earth what path to choose in fulfilling an occupational destiny. After high school, I went to college because it was a choice others wanted for me. Even though I had an academic scholarship, in my second year of college, after changing my major from business administration to history in the pursuit of a bachelor's degree, I found myself asking, "Why am I here?"

I left at the beginning of my junior year, married and became a mom. I stayed home with my daughter until she was four months old. At this time I saw an exciting commercial telling of how it would be great to get a nursing assistant certification from a local community college. However, once I went to the campus and spoke with the school's representative, he convinced me to go after the program for medical assistants stating it would only be one year longer than the curriculum for the nursing assistant. I would also gain more skill, knowledge and versatility. Choosing to be a medical assistant was a life –altering decision.

Medical assisting brings many rewards, but it is not an easy road to travel. This book is designed to help the medical assistant navigate the many challenges presented in the doctor's office.

The Doctor is in the House

IT IS ALWAYS an honor to work for a doctor. The acquisition of knowledge that brought him to the pinnacle of medicine commands respect.

I've worked with numerous doctors of all different types of dispositions. It is extremely helpful to the MA to first determine the personality of the doctor. Some doctors are a pleasure to work with even if there are endless challenges throughout the day. On the opposite end of the spectrum, you can stand on your head and do endless somersaults and still the doctor will look at you as it if it took an act of Congress to be passed for him to tolerate you. There are some doctors who are abusive. There is a difference between correction and insult.

I will be the first one to tell you that if you are facing abuse in the medical office whether it be from the doctor or other personnel-put in your two-weeks notice! You don't have to take it. I walked off one job in tears because I could no longer handle the unprofessional manner in which I was treated. I could not imagine two more weeks of this treatment. I have one credo that is known to everyone: "Treat everyone the way you want to be treated."

I take my job seriously. I've seen some critically ill people. On the days when I'm exhausted and I have one more patient to "bring back", I envision myself in the patient's shoes. How would I want to be treated? On more than one occasion I've been told by a patient that I'm the first person seen to smile in the office in a long time. Sometimes a smile can go further than an injection.

On occasion you can become attached to patients. Some instructors discourage being friendly with a patient. I say when you lose your ability to care, it's time to get out of the medical profession.

Formal Training or On-the-Job Training?

MY TRAINING BEGAN in the formal classroom setting. I had one year of training then I had to place the classroom on hold for years due to personal setbacks. Fortunately, I was able to use what I learned in that first year to get my foot in the door at a hospital cytology lab. The word cytology literally means the study of the cell. The course on Medical Terminology was priceless. It enabled me to speak very professionally in the lab.

In cytology, specimens are prepared by placing them on a slide or spinning the fluids down in a centrifuge in a special solution before placing the drops on the slide. The slide is then stained with coloring agents to make it easier for the pathologists to look at the slide through a microscope to determine if a disease process is occurring in a cell. Specifically, the doctor is looking for possible cancer cells or other diseases that can make a person acutely ill. Mainly fluids are studied in cytology, i.e. blood, urine or other fluids secreted by various systems of the body.

The other classes that I took that first crucial year in the classroom also included Anatomy and Physiology and courses in Phlebotomy. They were so invaluable to me as I learned the ropes of working in the lab. I was very fortunate to have thorough instructors who helped me to obtain my CPR and First Aid Certification and gave me practical experience with conducting basic lab tests-like erythrocyte (red blood cell) sedimentation rates which entails studying blood in a tube to see how fast the cells settle on the bottom indicating degrees of inflammation. More often than not it would be our own blood that was drawn while phlebotomy was being taught.

Many medical assistants are hired without formal training. If this is the case in your situation, I would recommend the purchase of books on the specific specialty of your employment. I especially recommend finding a book on medical terminology. Do not hesitate to ask questions. I remember the first time I worked in a pediatric office I was so embarrassed to ask another assistant to help me strengthen my blood pressure skills. At first she kind of gave me a strange look like, " I can't believe you don't know how to do this." I was too embarrassed to say I only practiced a few times in class. Now, I revel in the fact that I can take a manual blood pressure reading with very little effort. I could probably do it in my sleep. I actually prefer manual blood pressure readings over digital. I've learned that if the blood pressure cuff is too small, especially in adult readings, a false elevated reading could result. Also, with digital thermometers the battery could be low resulting in a false reading or no reading.

I did return to formal training to complete my degree and study for the certification test. I cannot describe the excitement I felt when I opened the envelope and beheld a passing score! Certification is not a requirement for most jobs, but if you decide to pursue it you must complete a degree in medical assisting. Certification may be the deciding factor on whether or not you land the job.

I have seen some wonderful MA's in action who were never formally trained, and I have seen some mediocre medical assistants who were formally trained. Classroom instruction gives you the theory behind various procedures that are performed in the doctor's office, but experience is the best teacher. However, if you have both, you will be bring the best of both worlds to your career. If I had to do it all over again, I would still find myself in the classroom first.

I want to tell you of the pitfalls and the joys I have encountered in the medical office. Hopefully, my trek will help you to expect the unexpected and navigate the medical office with confidence.

Not Enough Hands To Go Around

IN THIS DAY and age of economic trials, an MA can almost always expect to feel the stress of needing an extra pair of hands. Some offices cannot afford to hire more than a certain number of MAs. Some offices can afford it but may underestimate the value of a medical assistant believing that the status quo is sufficient even though it presents a strain on the personnel on board.

If an MA is absent in a situation where there aren't enough hands to go around to begin with, other staff can help close the gap by the reassignment of tasks. Usually, the situation turns out okay. However, if the MA is expected to do double the work, it can make for a very long day.

Medical assistants need to know that the job is an integral part of medical care. Giving a patient a prescribed vitamin B 12 injection that prevents a patient from losing his equilibrium, taking a chest x-ray that helps the doctor make a more definitive diagnosis and/or giving a nebulizer treatment so a patient with bronchitis can breathe more easily are only a few examples of the importance of MAs in the medical office.

MAs work under the supervision of doctors and nurses. There is nothing better than working right next to a nurse to accomplish the goal of helping a patient feel better. For example, I may be performing an electrocardiogram while a nurse may be hooking up a machine for the same patient to assess if the patient is accumulating too much fluid leading to edema in the limbs or around the heart. Also, if there is a wheelchair-bound patient that needs an x-ray, the teamwork comes into play again when one person makes sure the patient is held up while the other person snaps the x-ray. It results in a feeling of accomplishment for the whole team.

These are the element s of the job that keep me coming back again and again. It's hard to work if there aren't enough employees, but if the employees who are there are working as a team, it's amazing how the morale can be maintained with goal after goal being met throughout the day.

Personality and Time Management

THERE ARE PERSONALITY surveys that tell you what type of personality is best suited to a certain career. The bottom line for the MA profession is caring about people. If you have a passion for compassion and you follow through with the completion of assignments, you will shine like the sun in the field because the sky is the limit to what you can achieve.

Also, you have to have a personality. You should not act like a bump on a log. Incidentally, one aspect of the medical field caught me completely by surprise. This is the aspect of speed. I have been accused at various times of being too slow working up a patient which includes taking vital signs, going over medications and writing down symptoms.

However, you will encounter patients who are hard to tear yourself away from in a timely manner without being rude. You may ask a patient what the reason for the visit is and, all of a sudden, the person starts telling you what seems to be a life story. You have to know how to quickly question a patient to get a clear and concise answer because guess what? Time is money, and if the doctor determines you are taking too much time with the patient he will feel like you are compromising his time and funds.

I believe I am better than I used to be but sometimes I still encounter a patient whom as I am listening I know that a possible reprimand is coming my way for staying too long in the patient's room. Very rarely, even a doctor recognizes a patient who is hard to get away from because of details given that bear no relevance to the immediate symptoms.

When this occurs the doctor may ask for what is known as a rescue. A nurse or medical assistant may enter the room after a certain amount of time and summon the doctor out of the room. This is the truth and occurs especially if the doctor's schedule is double-booked in some spots during the day.

The point is for the doctor to stay on schedule. I try not to obviously rush the patient, but I also try to keep in mind that the longer I stay in a patient's room, the longer the doctor has to wait to talk to the patient or perform a possible procedure. The financial bottom line is always affected by time. If you need help getting a patient worked up in a timely manner, do not hesitate to ask another medical assistant or a nurse for help. Don't wait until your eyes glaze over before recognizing that too much time has elapsed.

Notation! Notation! Notation!

IT IS A general saying in the medical field that if a notation is not made then a prescribed procedure or statement did not take place. Medical records are subject to subpoena. If you give an injection, notate it along with the injection site and lot number of the medicine.

If you call in a prescription to the pharmacy, notate it along with the name of the pharmacy tech and/or pharmacist. I cannot stress this enough!!!!!!!!!! If anything can be notated, do it. It will legally protect you and the physician. It will also assure the physician that you are thorough. Notation also helps with medical billing. If there is a question as to whether or not a patient had an in-office procedure, the chart can be checked to confirm it. Some practices have a procedure log. It is a safeguard against an accusation that the job was not done. Verification is done through the written trail you leave.

If you spoke to someone at another office or lab, it is a good policy to notate the request and the person you spoke to at the facility. It is not unusual to be accused by the other office personnel of not making the telephone call or sending an urgent fax (by the way, it is a good idea to place the fax confirmation in the chart), but when you can give them the name of the person you spoke to, it usually dispels the confusion. Notate the date and time of the call. If your office uses electronic medical records, the date and time stamp will automatically occur when you save the information. If there is a delay in getting critical information and you let the physician know you spoke to the office several times giving specific names, then the physician will most likely call with the results coming through post haste with your credibility in tact.

Weighty Matters

DON'T UNDERESTIMATE THE importance of taking weight. Unless otherwise told, take the weight *everytime!* Even if the patient came in the day before, it is of the utmost importance that you take the weight, especially if the person is acutely ill with vomiting and diarrhea. Weight loss (a possible sign of anemia, cancer, or other disease process) or weight gain (a possible sign that the patient is accumulating fluid which may be indicative of heart disease and may also be indicative of cancer, i.e., thoracentesis fluid -chest fluid- specifically pleural fluid produced by the lungs and/or paracentesis/peritoneal fluid -abdominal fluid- may be an ominous sign of cancer) should be duly noted.

If the patient refuses to have a weight taken, you cannot force the issue. Always remember that patients have rights. Again, just notate that the patient refused to step on the scale. You cannot coerce a patient to follow a doctor's order. You may be accused of assault.

Some patients are wheel-chair bound. Again, notate this information in the chart so that someone coming behind you the next day realizes this fact and does not think you forgot to get the weight. Also, some patients may have weakness, dizziness or confusion which may actually make it dangerous for a weight to be taken.

Outside of the aforementioned exceptions, please make sure the weight is taken. A medical assistant who had forgotten to take the weight was released from the externship site by the physician. Thankfully, another site was quickly found. I, myself, did not take a weight once when I was a pediatric medical assistant, mistakenly thinking that it was the same patient I had weighed the previous day. I found out through another doctor in the practice that the doctor I was assigned to was practically livid. You can believe that after that episode I take weight without exception.

Why Medical Assisting?

IN WORKING AT many doctor's offices, I've been asked the question often, " Hi, are you the new nurse?" Many people are confused by the title and role of the medical assistant. Many medical assistants don't correct patients when they are referred to as nurses. I, on the other hand, take every opportunity to say, "No, I'm not a nurse, but my job is just as important."

A medical assistant is someone who is trained to "work patients up"-getting vital signs, accurate current patient medication lists and a concise description of the reason for the visit. Blood and other specimens may be obtained. Electrocardiograms may be performed and injections may be given by the medical assistant.

The medical assistant may also work in the administrative department-getting preauthorizations for medical procedures, checking in patients, answering the telephones and making sure co-pays are collected and that the insurance companies are billed correctly. These are actually only a few of the duties of the medical assistant.

A medical assistant is a great communicator and is able to multitask with an aptitude for science and a deep compassion and respect for others. The field is very rewarding and at times can be very intense. Not only will being a medical assistant make a difference in the lives of other people but it will also make a difference in your life. You cannot touch another person's life without being affected in profound ways. This career really helps you to keep your life in perspective, especially when you are assisting acutely ill patients. I chose medical assisting because of the benefits and never looked back. Facilitating patient care is very fulfilling for me.

An exceptional medical assistant will place the patient at ease so that the doctor and the patient can communicate without the normal anxiet that is felt immediately by the patient when entering the doctor's office.

Take a Breather!

MEDICAL ASSISTING CAN be very stressful at times. You may be great at multitasking but some days may be better than others. Some days *one* task can pull hard on your coping mechanisms. On those days, as soon as you are able to do it, take a breather. You may be rescued by the arrival of a lunch break where someone else will take over the job you are doing until you get back from your break or you may need to ask for help from another MA or nurse.

If you have a type A (undercover workaholic) personality like I do, asking for help can be very humbling. However, in a medical office you have to ask for help on occasion. Don't feel bad about it! If someone arrives for a procedure like hooking up a Holter heart monitor but you have a patient waiting just for a flu shot-ask for backup.

If you don't ask for help you run the risk of making a patient wait unnecessarily. Believe me, the physician does not want to see empty rooms and if there is a waiting area full of patients but you have become bogged down with one, reprimands will occur if reinforcements are not called in immediately.

The goal is to provide excellent patient care. Efficient patient care is a part of the equation. Patients who are made to wait may not return, regardless of the reason. Sometimes an emergency situation arises in which the doctor has to rush to the hospital. In this scenario, informing the patient of what has occurred generally helps so that the patient has the opportunity to reschedule the appointment.

One of the ways I cope with a hectic day is to leave the premises during lunch. I don't have to leave the building everyday, but if I don't on the days when everyone needs everything yesterday then I run the risk of feeling burnt out. If you only have a half hour for lunch, go to the store and pick up something healthy like a tuna fish snack pack and fruit juice. If you have an hour (what a luxury!), you can possibly go to a restaurant with a book, but be wary of a five-course meal at lunch that may leave you too sleepy to get through the rest of the day without being miserable.

After a stressful day, take care of you. I have yet to go to a spa for a massage, but relaxing can be easy. I make sure I walk around the local lake at least once a week. It does wonders for resolving my stress levels and it builds stamina. Aromatherapy or simple meditation also helps. If your job has paid time off days, put in for a vacation. Knowing that you have an extended break on the horizon helps most stressful situations at work. Get a manicure/pedicure complete with the back massage chair! It will take you into another stratosphere! Knowing how to take a break is key to occupational longevity as a medical assistant.

Mum is Definitely Not The Word

MANY PATIENTS WILL give you more than enough information to write a clear, concise statement for the physician regarding symptoms even before the physician enters the room. However, some patients state that certain medications have been discontinued but they will say that they don't want the doctor to know or maybe they did not complete all of their physical therapy regimen.

It is your ethical responsibility as an MA to make sure the doctor knows if a patient has been non-compliant with orders. If the doctor is not informed of the situation, a patient's health could be compromised and you could be fired. You are the liason between the physician and the patient. You'd be amazed at how lab tests will let the physician know anyway if the patient is taking the prescribed medication. If you are privy to the knowledge that the patient is not taking the medicine-notate it. It can save the patient's life!

Also, if you suspect the patient has been abused, you are legally obligated to report it. Reporting abuse to the physician who will report it to the proper authorities can also save a life. Besides, it is the humane thing to do, especially when children and elderly patients are involved.. Choosing to keep quiet can only cause harm so please *do the right thing.*

Administrative or Clinical?

I WILL BE the first one to say that I take my hat off to *anyone* who works "up front" in a medical office. I have worked as a medical receptionist and I have done physician referrals along with answering telephones, confirming appointments and verifying insurance benefits. Those were really long days! The administrative medical assistant bears the brunt of patients who are irritated because of seemingly endless wait times or because of insurance issues. They also have to deal with patients who call wanting immediate action for non-emergency situations that from the patients perspective are emergencies but are in fact situations that don't warrant immediate attention. Then there are the actual emergencies in which patients must be seen and placed in time slots that may be double or triple booked.

Thorough training allows the medical assistant to help out "up front" (administrative/clerical) or "in the back" (clinical). Sometimes the medical assistant has to do both if the office is small. My strength lies in the clinical area. On the days I have to help out up front I know I should be earning hazardous duty pay. It takes a special kind of person to juggle the demands of working the front desk or being on the telephone with an insurance company for hours trying to get pre-authorization for a hospital procedure. On the other hand, there is more room for promotion when one does administrative/clerical assisting. It is not unheard of for medical assistants who have a strong gift for administrative/clerical assisting to be promoted to supervisory positions.

I also know many medical assistants who would not want to deal with collecting specimens because they may experience nausea assisting with certain procedures. I remember asking an administrative medical assisting instructor with years of wonderful experience as a supervisor why she choose the administrative path.She said that she actually went to school to train for a clinical job and was in the home stretch to graduation but when it actually came to doing the hands on procedures, she stated that she did not have the stomach for it. You never really know what life has in store for you. It was many years ago that I walked through the door to apply for a hospital position but turned around before I reached the human resources door. Somehow I smelled what I termed at the time as that "hospital" smell. It is hard to fathom that this situation actually happened to me and that I somehow overcame it. Life is just filled with surprises, twists and turns.

I learned a great deal from the administrative instructor on understanding coding but I sure was glad when I finished that class. The clinical aspect of medical assisting is a joy for me. It is just a passion. Just ask anyone of my co-workers how many times I have volunteered to do an electrocardiogram and/or chest x-ray as they were on their way to performing the procedures.

As previously mentioned, the act of performing a manual

blood pressure reading has been the most valuable task I have learned. Detecting an accurate elevated blood pressure reading can be the difference between life and death as well as accurately detecting an extremely low blood pressure reading. A reading that is consistently high or low can point to several diagnoses and coupled with other presenting symptoms can result in the physician formulating an effective treatment plan.

Other clinical procedures I have assisted in performing include one-touch glucose readings, lancing of cysts, assisting with stitch removal, assisting with stress tests, giving screening tests for strep throat and the flu. I've also done phlebotomy which is definitely not my forte. If I cannot see your veins from across the street than more often times than not I'll grab someone from the lab. One day ,though, I am claiming that I will be able to get the vein the *first* time on everyone(Well, okay, I have the right to dream). Fortunately, I have not had to do a lot of phlebotomy. As the American Medical Association (AAMA) states, medical assisting is a very versatile profession.

In the fifteen years I have practiced medical assisting, I have seen the medical assistant go from just being able to take vital signs to having more involvement in patient care. The scope of the role depends on the office in which you work. Whether administrative ,clerical, or clinical, the medical assistant is truly the cornerstone of the medical office.

Why Certification?

MEDICAL ASSISTANTS ARE not required to be certified. However, certification lets your potential employer know that you are competent with more that the basic knowledge of medicine. It lets them know that you at least have the core skills needed for success in the medical office.

I received my medical training in the classroom and on the job. I started my medical training in the classroom, but I left formal training for many years. I was going through a divorce and decided that I needed to work full time to support my daughter. It was fifteen years before I made it back to the classroom. That is why it is so imperative to stay in school because once you leave it seems almost impossible to return once family and work demands pile up.

I never had trouble finding a job in the field because I did complete a full year of the two-year curriculum which included medical terminology and phlebotomy along with a hosts of hands-on information regarding lab tests and the required anatomy and physiology courses.

It always bothered me that I did not finish my degree in

medical assisting. It bothered me even more that I was not certified even though certification is not a prerequisite for the hiring of most medical assistants. I hold myself up to a higher level and I always wandered if I could attain it. When my daughter started college I started purchasing expensive medical assisting certification preparatory books, but I did not have the attention span to sit down and go through all of the practice tests on my own without professional guidance.

I decided one day to drive to my former school on a whim just to gather information. One week later, I was in the classroom. It was the best thing I ever did for my career! I had forgotten that I did have excellent grades all those years ago and with no small degree of anxiety, I was determined to maintain my 4.0 average. Now, for many years I was under the impression that I could take the certification even though I had not finished the degree because of my years of experience. I was really wrong about that part! It is a good thing I decided to go back to school or else I never would have become certified.

My teachers were great and gave me the guidance I needed not only to sharpen my clinical skills of phlebotomy and performing various lab tests like blood typing, erythrocyte sedimentation rates and calculations for intravenous fluids and injections but they also helped to give me the discipline I needed to study for my examinations.

At the end of the curriculum I had to do a 300 hour unpaid externship. It wasn't easy. As a matter of fact, I was laid off as a neurological medical assistant because I was told there were no part-time positions available even though I was given a promise that the staff would work with me. I had only ten week left to finish my degree. I was devastated! I successfully applied for unemployment which has to be one of the most humiliating experiences one has to endure if you in fact want to work. However, I pulled myself together and finished my externship. Talk about challenging circumstances! I knew, though that the Lord didn't bring me this far to leave me!

It was one of the hardest periods in my life because the neurology position actually was the biggest inspiration for my decision to go after certification. I wanted certification so that it could help me be the best I could be professionally for this particular job. One is never prepared to be blindsided but there is a silver lining around every cloud!

As a neurological medical assistant, I could not fully use my degree as I only took vital signs and called other offices for medical records. Now, as a cardiac medical assistant, I get to perform a plethora of procedures I only dreamed of before I received my associates degree.

I graduated *summa cum laude* and I shall never forget that day. I would not trade my classroom instruction for anything in this world!

Taking the certification examination was incredibly hard. The test was 3-4 hours long and included questions covering clinical, administrative and general knowledge areas. I had to bring my classroom instruction together with my on-the-job training to get through the test.

I was on pins and needles until I received the results. There are few words in the English language as beautiful as the word "PASSED!" So now I have my certification on my desk area at work and I have my degree hanging in my bedroom so that when I wake up it's one of the first things I see. There is nothing like the feeling of accomplishment it gives you and the message it gives the world: " I am competent and ready to take on the task at hand."

You Get As Much As You Give

I LEARN SO much from patients every day. It is such an honor to serve them. Many times I get so busy I meet myself coming and going, but I try to take the time to listen to what the patients are saying in addition to making sure I painstakingly work the patient up. I cannot tell you how many recipes, advice on gardening, where to go for vacations and other valuable tidbits of information I have received that have enriched my life.

When I'm having a challenging day, it only takes one patient to turn it around. I've heard jokes that are funny and some that fall short of the humor mark, but it is inspiring to know that a person who is battling a health condition want to brighten another's day.

It's also great to work in an office and see someone often enough that you remember his or her name without getting it from the chart. It can be the little things that can make a big difference in a person's life. Sure there have been negative experiences, but I refuse to dwell on them and I certainly do not hold any grudges against those who choose to take out their frustrations on me on any given day. Life is just too full of promise to hold onto something that doesn't matter when one looks at the big picture. However, if I offend someone or make a mistake, I am quick to say that it's my fault and I try everything I can to make the situation better. Nobody's perfect.

Please remember to follow through with a patient. If you tell a patient you will call them back-do it. If you are getting a prior authorization so the patient's insurance will pay for a special medication and it will take a few days, please let the patient know you are working on the matter. Please be proactive. No one wants to feel as if someone has forgotten a problem. It's always fulfilling to hear "Thank You" once the task has been completed.

Health Concerns

ONE OF THE best advantages of working as a certified medical assistant is knowing that you have the most current medical knowledge right at hand. The resources can range from the latest technology for prescreening for abdominal aortic aneurysms to being informed of the most recent sample of the latest vaccination in the fight against pediatric cancer. With my family history of hyperlipidemia and pulmonary emboli deaths, it is not only academically beneficial to have access to this wealth of medical resources, but it is also personally lifesaving.

It is my responsibility to make sure my family members stay healthy. So I do not hesitate to keep a check on blood pressure readings and to make sure doctor's appointments are kept so that appropriate labs are drawn in a timely manner. Prevention is the key to a lifetime of good health. You always hear it but it is the truth: Getting regular checkups is the key to nipping medical crises in the bud.

It is easy to surf the web for answers, however, nothing beats actually having access to a physician's wisdom on a daily basis.

Is Medical Assisting Enough?

DURING THE PINNING ceremony before graduation, I was asked to give a speech to my fellow medical assistants poised on the brink of a promising career. As an older student, I had a maternal attitude towards my classmates.

In the speech, I assured them that they would do well in their careers and that at some point they may want to receive more "schooling". My main message was to let them know that it is okay to pursue other vocations, but not if they thought medical assisting was not enough. At one time, I wanted to go back to school to be a radiological technician-until I was taught to do chest x-rays as a medical assistant. I feel like I have the world at my fingertips as an MA.

Being a medical assistant may inspire you to go back to school to be a nurse or a physician's assistant or it may convince you to go all the way by going to medical school but, I would not leave the profession merely because of the thought that medical assisting is not enough.

I have also thought of returning to school to become an ultrasonographer because as a medical assistant I have cultivated a love of machines. In this scenario it is the love of the field of medicine and the desire for growth that drives me to consider returning to school. I would not go for the financial aspects because that alone would not be fulfilling for me. As a matter of fact if you decide to apply for medical school and told the interviewer you were applying for monetary gain, you application would be rejected immediately. It's not about the money. It's about the love of the medical field that underscores success in any area of medicine.

I once remember reading about an MA who hated the question: "Why don't you go back to school to be a nurse?" For her being an MA was more than enough. For me, at this point in time, it's more than enough. If I decided to go back to school it would be a natural progression. Most people, regardless of the career, will seek advancement at some stage. Medical assisting is an incredible stepping stone to any career in the medical field!

Good Evening Professors, Administrators, Distinguished Guests and My Fellow Medical Assistants!

I AM SO very proud of all of us who have made it this far. All of us have stories to tell of the trials, tribulations and accomplishments that brought us to this point. All of our stories are unique-mine included.

Fifteen years ago, I was blessed to have come to this university when it was South College-not quite as big as it is today, but just as valuable.

I know there are those of you who wonder whether or not it was worth it academically, financially or professionally. I am standing before you as proof that it is indeed worth it.

Fifteen years ago, I came here for one academic year. After that year I had to leave for personal reasons-but just that one academic year gave me what I needed to compete in the job market. The medical terminology, anatomy and physiology, phlebotomy and clinicals combined gave me the required foundation needed to thrive in the field.

However, it always bothered me that I never finished. It always bothered me that I didn't complete my Associate's Degree-that I didn't have CMA after my name-that I had to work twice as hard to prove to any given employer that I was competent ant a mistake was not make in hiring me.

Today, I am so close to reaching my goal that I could *shout* with anticipation!

You will encounter individuals who will tell you it is not enough to be a medical assistant-that you should go higher-and ofcourse, you should always try to better yourself-but not because you feel it is not enough. I assure you it is.

A medical assistant is the cornerstone of the doctor's office. The office cannot run efficiently without the talents of a medical assistant. I cannot even conceive of an office without one of us. We are the first ones to come in contact with the patient who is anxious and usually in pain, trying to make his or her way to the doctor. It is up to us to *listen* to the patient and to provide a safe, secure and confidential environment. It is up to us to provide the standard of care that each patient deserves and the standard of care we know we can give.

And when all else fails and you are weary, but you have one more patient between you and the end of the day, put yourself in that patient's shoes and you will have no problem with standard of care.

I appreciate all of my professors and the knowledge they have bestowed upon me. I want to give special thanks to Ms. Deborah Brinkman for helping to give me the courage I needed to be back in the classroom after all those years. Coming back to South University has been like coming back home.

I want to leave you with a quote from someone who has always inspired me. This person overcame very real obstacles to become a shining example of humanity. Her name was Helen Keller and I quote:

"Many people have the wrong idea of what constitutes true happiness. It's not attained through self gratification but fidelity to a worthy purpose." (Unquote)

I feel that medical assisting is for me that worthy purpose.

THANK YOU AND CONGRATULATIONS TO ALL OF US!

The speech given by the author at the pinning ceremony days before graduation in 2008. She was chosen to give the speech because of her 4.0 GPA.

AFTERWORD AND ACKNOWLEDGEMENTS

IT HAS BEEN some years since my graduation and my knowledge as a medical assistant has grown by leaps and bounds. My passion for the field is just as strong. It is surprising the opportunities that present themselves on a daily basis. I want to say I have aged gracefully since my graduation but aging is not an easy road. I feel the exercise I get as a certified medical assistant keeps me young but I am proud to say that I am the grandmother of one born on Valentine's Day. How sweet is that? Xavier will probably be three at the time of the publication of this book and he lets me know that soon it will truly be time to pass the baton.

This book has been on the backburner for a long time. I almost turned the fire off from under it but it's funny how when something is meant to be it creates its own fire within you.

I want to give my wonderful husband, Pastor Elijah Gregory, credit for putting up with me as long as he has because I know

I can be quite the handful. Only with Grace have we been able to steadily continue down the aisle of matrimony.

I also want to thank my beloved brother, Johnny Wade, for providing a listening ear when I needed to rant and rave. God bless him for his patience.

I cannot close without giving due diligence and credit to Outskirts Press for publishing this book. They believed in me during a time when I did not believe in myself. The existence of this published work shows that all things are possible through Christ which strengthens us.

www.ingramcontent.com/pod-product-compliance
Lightning Source LLC
Chambersburg PA
CBHW021050180526
45163CB00005B/2363